HOW TO LOSE BELLY FAT QUICK

Michael J. Roberts

TABLE OF CONTENTS

INTRODUCTION

FRUITS AND VEGGIES

EXERCISE

REDUCING CALORIES

ADDING AN OPPOSITION BAND

AVOIDING CARBONATED BEVERAGES

AVOIDING GASSY AND ACIDIC FOODS

HAVING A DIET PLAN

KIND OF CALORIE

EXERCISE INSTRUCTION MANUAL

STABILITY BALL

THE ESSENCE OF MUSCLE

WORKOUT 1

CARDIO

CARDIO ROUTINE

METABOLIC SYNDROME

REAL FOODS

FOOT LIFTING

CARDIO EXERCISE

WORKING OUT YIELDS BETTER RESULT

RESEARCH AT SACRAMENTO STATE COLLEGE

SUBSTITUTING FOODS TO RESERVE ENERGY

POSITIVE EFFECT OF USING THE STABILITY BALL

THE INVERT CRUNCH

THE ROCK AND ROLL WORKOUT

WORKOUT 2

THE PIKE

MODIFYING YOUR EATING HABIT

INTRODUCTION

Paunch fat is additional tummy fat encompassing the organs in your pelvis. There are three kinds of fat:

triglycerides (the paunch that circulates in your blood), epidermal fat (the layer specifically underneath the skin's surface), and visceral fat (perilous paunch fat).

FRUITS AND VEGGIES

To begin with, you need to have an adjusted calorie intake. One recommendation is to "eat around the exterior of the supermarket." That is, do not go into the islands where all the prepared nourishment is. Instep, eat parcels of new natural products and vegetables as well as a direct sum of incline meat and moo fat dairy items. Bulk up with characteristic nutrients like grains and vegetables.

EXERCISE

Perfect way">The most perfect way to do high-impact work out is tall escalated interim preparation. This is often where you are doing a two-minute diminutive burst of movement at the most serious level you're competent at, followed by three minutes of direct action. Rehash the cycle.

REDUCING CALORIES

Inevitably, you have got to diminish your kilocalories. You need to eat 500 occasional kilocalories than you'd otherwise to preserve your weight. A 30-year-old man who is 5'10 and weighs 180 pounds needs almost 2700 kilocalories to preserve his weight. He ought to eat, as there are 2200 calories on this program.

ADDING AN OPPOSITION BAND

An opposition band takes the work out and makes it additionally serious. You ought to likely begin out doing the developments without any sort of opposition at all to help you seem like you're losing belly fat. And once the straightforward development gets a little bit simpler at that point, include a resistance band or a few other types of resistance to take it up a notch. Adding resistance to nearly any development outlined to make your paunch look less fat will essentially make things happen faster.

AVOIDING CARBONATED BEVERAGES

Dodging brunches that are aerated and full of sugar, like pop, can help decrease your stomach as well. Whereas you might not be shedding stomach fat to make it smaller, it'll be less full of either nourishment or the gases caused by carbonation and will show up smaller.

AVOIDING GASSY AND ACIDIC FOODS

You'll lose fat somewhere else around your body, but not in your paunch. A few diets claim to allow you a level paunch, but it's fair conventional weight misfortune and maybe a few nourishment choices that get rid of stomach bloat. Eating nourishments that aren't gassy or acidic can help make your stomach appear smaller since you decrease the gas and bloating that you simply might have.

HAVING A DIET PLAN

So, one of the component of the fastest way to lose belly fat is to come up with a healthy eating plan. Usually, an eating arrangement is for life; not a few crazes eat less. After you lose weight, you compound the belly fat issue since you lose weight in other ranges, but you put it back on within the stomach zone to begin with. So, making an alter in your slim down on a changeless premise is key. You're creating a way of life, not going on a transitory slim down.

KIND OF CALORIE

Your slim down ought to be concerned not as much with the whole number of calories as with the sorts of calories. You wish to require at least 1 gram of protein per day for each pound you weigh. You, too, require a few fats in your daily calorie intake. A slim-down of 30:20:50 within the proportion of protein: fat: Carbohydrates make a lot of sense for an overweight lady who needs the speediest way to lose belly fat. Angle oils are the finest kind of fat for this reason.

EXERCISE INSTRUCTION MANUAL

When you buy a ball, it arrives with instructions for utilizing it in various exercises.

There is usually a diagram showing what you need to do.

Therefore, we will discuss only some of them here.

STABILITY BALL

To begin with, to shed paunch fat, you wish to purchase a solidity ball. These retail for almost $30 in a retail clothing store. Most ladies will want a 22-inch ball. On the off chance that you're under 5'1, purchase the 18-inch, and in the event that you're over 5'8, go for the 26-inch.

THE ESSENCE OF MUSCLE

Muscle is vital, but it may not assist you in really losing weight, at least not according to your scale; it all depends on how well you lose stomach fat and how much muscle tissue you build up. The reason is typically that muscle weighs more than the same volume of fat. Don't let that panic you away from the solidity ball, although typically, it's a great thing! Whether you need to see superiority or diminish your chance for certain illnesses, what you're truly attempting to do is be more advantageous. Muscle tissue will not, as it were, make you see way better, but it'll also burn a few calories while you're at rest.

WORKOUT 1

One prevalent schedule that can get rid of 500 kilocalories in a single period has you working out for 3 minutes, picking up the intensity for 3 minutes, stretching yourself as difficult as you'll be able for two minutes, and at that point, abating down for 3 minutes, followed by pushing yourself for another 2 minutes. Rehash this for a total of 45 minutes, some time ago, while doing a 2-minute cool-down period.

<u>CARDIO</u>

Aerophilic workouts are also crucial to this plan.

To lessen baby paunch fat, try doing her heart-healthy 45-minute workout at least three times a week.

This includes brisk walking, jogging, cycling, and using cardio machines at the gym.

CARDIO ROUTINE

At that point, commence building up a cardio schedule. You ought to be doing heart-sound exercises at least four times every week. It appeared that dieters who strolled for 50 minutes four successive times every week lost about twice as much belly fat as those who decreased their kilocalories.

METABOLIC SYNDROME

Metabolic sickness may be a sickness that includes rising blood sugar, heightened hemoglobin weight, and an inflated body weight. Persons with a bit of belly fat tend to endure this more frequently. It's not known if the disorder is present to begin with and causes the stomach fat, or if individuals who have more belly fat are more inclined to the disorder.

REAL FOODS

Choosing foods that are part of an entire diet and dodging profoundly handled diets can offer help in diminishing bloating and any swelling that could be contributing to a bigger stomach. Diets that center on genuine nourishment and entire nourishment can certainly offer assistance with this.

FOOT LIFTING

Utilize the same position as you did for the situated walk. This time, rather than employing a walking movement, you're progressing to lift one foot off the floor and, after that, hold it within the discussion for 5 to 10 seconds, sometimes recently exchanging to the other foot.

CARDIO EXERCISE

Whereas the ball is central to this arrangement, it isn't the only component. The fastest way to lose belly fat, too, includes doing 50 minutes of cardio at least three times a week. You need to warm up for three minutes, and after that, interchange between three minutes of a customary-paced workout and two minutes of pushing yourself as hard as you'll. Cool down for two minutes at the conclusion. You'll do any kind of heart-sound workout, counting strolling, running, cycling, or employing a cardio machine at the exercise center.

WORKING OUT YIELDS BETTER RESULT

It is, be that as it may, the workout that will offer assistance in recoiling the stomach more than the slim down. But you might discover that if you've been eating generously for a long time and you go on a great eating arrangement, your paunch will appear a little bit absent. That's essentially because your stomach is not full and bloated from as much nourishment or off-base sorts of nourishment.

RESEARCH AT SACRAMENTO STATE COLLEGE

A study at Sacramento State College found that individuals who utilized steadiness balls to lose stomach fat had created twice the number of muscle strands as those who did typical crunches. As you'll see, this will help you lose stomach fat rapidly, so you'll need to induce one.

SUBSTITUTING FOODS TO RESERVE ENERGY

Finding ways to diminish calories for a brief period is less demanding than you might imagine. For instance, making your latte with skim milk instead of entire milk saves 120 calories. You'll be able to live with that for two weeks, won't you? Other swaps incorporate eating popped popcorn rather than potato chips (spares 95 calories) and substituting ½ glass of cut strawberries and ½ container of fat-free vanilla yogurt for your conventional "fruit on the bottom" yogurt container (spares 105 calories). Make 4 to 5 of these substitutions a day, and you're on your way to losing infant paunch fat.

POSITIVE EFFECT OF USING THE STABILITY BALL

Your body will always be attempting to adjust itself when you're using the ball. Chances are you won't indeed take note of a part of these movements, but you'll be beyond any doubt that the ball is working. Whereas there's still more research to be done, at least one bunch of analysts has found that employing a soundness ball amid certain workouts can about double the number of muscle filaments within the focused zone.

THE INVERT CRUNCH

There will be several exercises within the manual that come with the soundness ball, but I want to highlight some here that are especially supportive after you need to lose a child's stomach fat. The primary is the invert crunch. Lying on your back, press your legs into the ball and lift it 3 to 6 inches off the floor. Hold it for one moment, then lower and rehash.

THE ROCK AND ROLL WORKOUT

The second is the shake and roll. Get on your knees and put your elbows on the ball. At that point, lift your body until you're on your tippy toes at a 45-degree projection to the earth. Sustain this position for one moment, unwind, and rehash.

WORKOUT 2

Sit on the bare base as if you were doing curl-ups, but raise the body about halfway up.

First, learn the correct form to avoid injury.

Keep your face facing the ceiling and use your abdominal strength, not your neck or back, to lift yourself.

If you use it on your back, it won't work on your stomach.

THE PIKE

The moment is named the Pike, and it's one of the more complicated artifices you'll do with the steady ball. You ought to lie on the ball, and your legs ought to be along with the ball beneath your thighs. Keep your legs straight, contract your abs, and lift your hips toward the ceiling, rolling the ball to the shins. Hold for one moment, and after that, lower.

MODIFYING YOUR EATING HABIT

The final step is to alter your eating habits.

Try to eat 500 more occasional kilocalories than you need to retain your weight.

For example, an active 28-year-old woman who is 5 feet 10 inches tall and weighs 130 pounds will need 2,400 kilocalories to maintain her weight.

During her two weeks on this program, she must eat only 1,900 calories.

Made in United States
North Haven, CT
20 April 2025